# My Medical Binder

**This Binder Belongs To:**

**Name:**
_____

**Contact Information:**
_____

"My Medical Binder" Copyright 2013, Chelsea Makela. All Rights Reserved.

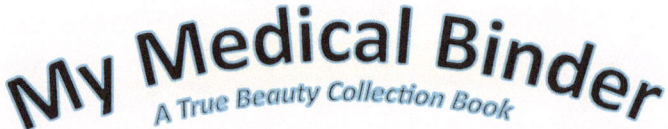

Notice that "All rights reserved".
Copyright 2013, Chelsea Makela.
All Rights Reserved.

This book is meant to be used for journaling and personal purposes only it does not qualify as medical or nutritional advice. Please speak to/consult a medical professional(s) to verify and check any medical needs and/or conditions, services/advice/information

# My Contacts & Information:

**Name:**
_____
_____

**Patient ID Number:**
_____
_____

**Age:**
_____
_____

**Contact Number:**
_____
_____

**Emergency Contact:**
_____
_____

**My Doctor (s) Name/Contact:**
_____
_____

**Medications I Am Taking:**
_____
_____

**Insurance Name/Number/Contact:**
_____
_____

**Allergies & Things EMT/Emergency Personnel Need To Know:**
_____
_____

"My Medical Binder" Copyright 2013, Chelsea Makela. All Rights Reserved.

# My Schedule

"My Medical Binder"
Copyright 2013, Chelsea Makela. All Rights Reserved.

| Sun. | Mon. | Tues. | Wed. | Thurs. | Fri. | Sat. |
|------|------|-------|------|--------|------|------|
|      |      |       |      |        |      |      |
|      |      |       |      |        |      |      |
|      |      |       |      |        |      |      |
|      |      |       |      |        |      |      |

"My Medical Binder" Copyright 2013, Chelsea Makela. All Rights Reserved.

|  Sun. | Mon. | Tues. | Wed. | Thurs. | Fri. | Sat. |
|---|---|---|---|---|---|---|
|  |  |  |  |  |  |  |
|  |  |  |  |  |  |  |
|  |  |  |  |  |  |  |
|  |  |  |  |  |  |  |

"My Medical Binder" Copyright 2013, Chelsea Makela. All Rights Reserved.

| Sun. | Mon. | Tues. | Wed. | Thurs. | Fri. | Sat. |
|------|------|-------|------|--------|------|------|
|      |      |       |      |        |      |      |
|      |      |       |      |        |      |      |
|      |      |       |      |        |      |      |
|      |      |       |      |        |      |      |

"My Medical Binder" Copyright 2013, Chelsea Makela. All Rights Reserved.

|  Sun. | Mon. | Tues. | Wed. | Thurs. | Fri. | Sat. |
|---|---|---|---|---|---|---|
|  |  |  |  |  |  |  |
|  |  |  |  |  |  |  |
|  |  |  |  |  |  |  |
|  |  |  |  |  |  |  |

"My Medical Binder" Copyright 2013, Chelsea Makela. All Rights Reserved.

| Sun. | Mon. | Tues. | Wed. | Thurs. | Fri. | Sat. |
|------|------|-------|------|--------|------|------|
|      |      |       |      |        |      |      |
|      |      |       |      |        |      |      |
|      |      |       |      |        |      |      |
|      |      |       |      |        |      |      |

"My Medical Binder" Copyright 2013, Chelsea Makela. All Rights Reserved.

| Sun. | Mon. | Tues. | Wed. | Thurs. | Fri. | Sat. |
|------|------|-------|------|--------|------|------|
|      |      |       |      |        |      |      |
|      |      |       |      |        |      |      |
|      |      |       |      |        |      |      |
|      |      |       |      |        |      |      |

"My Medical Binder" Copyright 2013, Chelsea Makela. All Rights Reserved.

| Sun. | Mon. | Tues. | Wed. | Thurs. | Fri. | Sat. |
|------|------|-------|------|--------|------|------|
|      |      |       |      |        |      |      |
|      |      |       |      |        |      |      |
|      |      |       |      |        |      |      |
|      |      |       |      |        |      |      |

"My Medical Binder" Copyright 2013, Chelsea Makela. All Rights Reserved.

| Sun. | Mon. | Tues. | Wed. | Thurs. | Fri. | Sat. |
|------|------|-------|------|--------|------|------|
|      |      |       |      |        |      |      |
|      |      |       |      |        |      |      |
|      |      |       |      |        |      |      |
|      |      |       |      |        |      |      |

"My Medical Binder" Copyright 2013, Chelsea Makela. All Rights Reserved.

| Sun. | Mon. | Tues. | Wed. | Thurs. | Fri. | Sat. |
|------|------|-------|------|--------|------|------|
|      |      |       |      |        |      |      |
|      |      |       |      |        |      |      |
|      |      |       |      |        |      |      |
|      |      |       |      |        |      |      |

"My Medical Binder" Copyright 2013, Chelsea Makela. All Rights Reserved.

|  Sun. | Mon. | Tues. | Wed. | Thurs. | Fri. | Sat. |
|---|---|---|---|---|---|---|
|  |  |  |  |  |  |  |
|  |  |  |  |  |  |  |
|  |  |  |  |  |  |  |
|  |  |  |  |  |  |  |

"My Medical Binder" Copyright 2013, Chelsea Makela. All Rights Reserved.

| Sun. | Mon. | Tues. | Wed. | Thurs. | Fri. | Sat. |
|------|------|-------|------|--------|------|------|
|      |      |       |      |        |      |      |
|      |      |       |      |        |      |      |
|      |      |       |      |        |      |      |
|      |      |       |      |        |      |      |

"My Medical Binder" Copyright 2013, Chelsea Makela. All Rights Reserved.

|  Sun. | Mon. | Tues. | Wed. | Thurs. | Fri. | Sat. |
| --- | --- | --- | --- | --- | --- | --- |
|  |  |  |  |  |  |  |
|  |  |  |  |  |  |  |
|  |  |  |  |  |  |  |
|  |  |  |  |  |  |  |

"My Medical Binder" Copyright 2013, Chelsea Makela. All Rights Reserved.

| Sun. | Mon. | Tues. | Wed. | Thurs. | Fri. | Sat. |
|------|------|-------|------|--------|------|------|
|      |      |       |      |        |      |      |
|      |      |       |      |        |      |      |
|      |      |       |      |        |      |      |
|      |      |       |      |        |      |      |

"My Medical Binder" Copyright 2013, Chelsea Makela. All Rights Reserved.

# My Medication

"My Medical Binder"
Copyright 2013, Chelsea Makela. All Rights Reserved.

**Name of Medication:**
_____
_____

**Dosage:**
_____
_____

**How Often I Take It:**
_____
_____

**Time (s) To Take:**
_____
_____
_____
_____

**Things to Remember:**
_____
_____
_____
_____

**Signs To Watch For:**
_____
_____
_____
_____

**Doctor that Prescribed Medication:**
_____
_____

**Start/Stop Medication:**
_____
_____

**Name of Medication:**
_____
_____

**Dosage:**
_____
_____

**How Often I Take It:**
_____
_____

**Time (s) To Take:**
_____
_____
_____
_____

**Things to Remember:**
_____
_____
_____
_____

**Signs To Watch For:**
_____
_____
_____
_____

**Doctor that Prescribed Medication:**
_____
_____

**Start/Stop Medication:**
_____
_____

"My Medical Binder" Copyright 2013, Chelsea Makela. All Rights Reserved.

| Name of Medication: | Name of Medication: |
|---|---|
| _____ | _____ |
| _____ | _____ |
| Dosage: | Dosage: |
| _____ | _____ |
| _____ | _____ |
| How Often I Take It: | How Often I Take It: |
| _____ | _____ |
| _____ | _____ |
| Time (s) To Take: | Time (s) To Take: |
| _____ | _____ |
| _____ | _____ |
| _____ | _____ |
| _____ | _____ |
| Things to Remember: | Things to Remember: |
| _____ | _____ |
| _____ | _____ |
| _____ | _____ |
| _____ | _____ |
| Signs To Watch For: | Signs To Watch For: |
| _____ | _____ |
| _____ | _____ |
| _____ | _____ |
| _____ | _____ |
| Doctor that Prescribed Medication: | Doctor that Prescribed Medication: |
| _____ | _____ |
| _____ | _____ |
| Start/Stop Medication: | Start/Stop Medication: |
| _____ | _____ |
| _____ | _____ |

"My Medical Binder" Copyright 2013, Chelsea Makela. All Rights Reserved.

| Name of Medication: | Name of Medication: |
|---|---|
| _____ | _____ |
| _____ | _____ |
| Dosage: | Dosage: |
| _____ | _____ |
| _____ | _____ |
| How Often I Take It: | How Often I Take It: |
| _____ | _____ |
| _____ | _____ |
| Time (s) To Take: | Time (s) To Take: |
| _____ | _____ |
| _____ | _____ |
| _____ | _____ |
| _____ | _____ |
| Things to Remember: | Things to Remember: |
| _____ | _____ |
| _____ | _____ |
| _____ | _____ |
| _____ | _____ |
| Signs To Watch For: | Signs To Watch For: |
| _____ | _____ |
| _____ | _____ |
| _____ | _____ |
| _____ | _____ |
| Doctor that Prescribed Medication: | Doctor that Prescribed Medication: |
| _____ | _____ |
| _____ | _____ |
| Start/Stop Medication: | Start/Stop Medication: |
| _____ | _____ |
| _____ | _____ |

"My Medical Binder" Copyright 2013, Chelsea Makela. All Rights Reserved.

| Name of Medication: | Name of Medication: |
|---|---|
| _____ | _____ |
| _____ | _____ |
| Dosage: | Dosage: |
| _____ | _____ |
| _____ | _____ |
| How Often I Take It: | How Often I Take It: |
| _____ | _____ |
| _____ | _____ |
| Time (s) To Take: | Time (s) To Take: |
| _____ | _____ |
| _____ | _____ |
| _____ | _____ |
| _____ | _____ |
| Things to Remember: | Things to Remember: |
| _____ | _____ |
| _____ | _____ |
| _____ | _____ |
| _____ | _____ |
| Signs To Watch For: | Signs To Watch For: |
| _____ | _____ |
| _____ | _____ |
| _____ | _____ |
| _____ | _____ |
| Doctor that Prescribed Medication: | Doctor that Prescribed Medication: |
| _____ | _____ |
| _____ | _____ |
| Start/Stop Medication: | Start/Stop Medication: |
| _____ | _____ |
| _____ | _____ |

"My Medical Binder" Copyright 2013, Chelsea Makela. All Rights Reserved.

**Name of Medication:**
_____
_____

**Dosage:**
_____
_____

**How Often I Take It:**
_____
_____

**Time (s) To Take:**
_____
_____
_____
_____

**Things to Remember:**
_____
_____
_____
_____

**Signs To Watch For:**
_____
_____
_____
_____

**Doctor that Prescribed Medication:**
_____
_____

**Start/Stop Medication:**
_____
_____

---

**Name of Medication:**
_____
_____

**Dosage:**
_____
_____

**How Often I Take It:**
_____
_____

**Time (s) To Take:**
_____
_____
_____
_____

**Things to Remember:**
_____
_____
_____
_____

**Signs To Watch For:**
_____
_____
_____
_____

**Doctor that Prescribed Medication:**
_____
_____

**Start/Stop Medication:**
_____
_____

"My Medical Binder" Copyright 2013, Chelsea Makela. All Rights Reserved.

| Name of Medication: | Name of Medication: |
|---|---|
| _____ | _____ |
| _____ | _____ |
| Dosage: | Dosage: |
| _____ | _____ |
| _____ | _____ |
| How Often I Take It: | How Often I Take It: |
| _____ | _____ |
| _____ | _____ |
| Time (s) To Take: | Time (s) To Take: |
| _____ | _____ |
| _____ | _____ |
| _____ | _____ |
| _____ | _____ |
| Things to Remember: | Things to Remember: |
| _____ | _____ |
| _____ | _____ |
| _____ | _____ |
| _____ | _____ |
| Signs To Watch For: | Signs To Watch For: |
| _____ | _____ |
| _____ | _____ |
| _____ | _____ |
| _____ | _____ |
| Doctor that Prescribed Medication: | Doctor that Prescribed Medication: |
| _____ | _____ |
| _____ | _____ |
| Start/Stop Medication: | Start/Stop Medication: |
| _____ | _____ |
| _____ | _____ |

"My Medical Binder" Copyright 2013, Chelsea Makela. All Rights Reserved.

**Name of Medication:**
_____
_____

 **Dosage:**
_____
_____

**How Often I Take It:**
_____
_____

**Time (s) To Take:**
_____
_____
_____

**Things to Remember:**
_____
_____
_____
_____

**Signs To Watch For:**
_____
_____
_____

**Doctor that Prescribed Medication:**
_____
_____

**Start/Stop Medication:**
_____
_____

**Name of Medication:**
_____
_____

 **Dosage:**
_____
_____

**How Often I Take It:**
_____
_____

**Time (s) To Take:**
_____
_____
_____

**Things to Remember:**
_____
_____
_____
_____

**Signs To Watch For:**
_____
_____
_____

**Doctor that Prescribed Medication:**
_____
_____

**Start/Stop Medication:**
_____
_____

"My Medical Binder" Copyright 2013, Chelsea Makela. All Rights Reserved.

| Name of Medication: | Name of Medication: |
| --- | --- |
| _____ | _____ |
| _____ | _____ |
| Dosage: | Dosage: |
| _____ | _____ |
| _____ | _____ |
| How Often I Take It: | How Often I Take It: |
| _____ | _____ |
| _____ | _____ |
| Time (s) To Take: | Time (s) To Take: |
| _____ | _____ |
| _____ | _____ |
| _____ | _____ |
| _____ | _____ |
| Things to Remember: | Things to Remember: |
| _____ | _____ |
| _____ | _____ |
| _____ | _____ |
| _____ | _____ |
| Signs To Watch For: | Signs To Watch For: |
| _____ | _____ |
| _____ | _____ |
| _____ | _____ |
| _____ | _____ |
| Doctor that Prescribed Medication: | Doctor that Prescribed Medication: |
| _____ | _____ |
| _____ | _____ |
| Start/Stop Medication: | Start/Stop Medication: |
| _____ | _____ |
| _____ | _____ |

"My Medical Binder" Copyright 2013, Chelsea Makela. All Rights Reserved.

# My Medicine Log

"My Medical Binder"
Copyright 2013, Chelsea Makela. All Rights Reserved.

# My Medicine Log

| Medicine Name: | Time to Take: AM/PM | Dose: | With or Without Food? |
|---|---|---|---|
| | | | |
| | | | |
| | | | |
| | | | |
| | | | |
| | | | |
| | | | |
| | | | |
| | | | |
| | | | |
| | | | |

"My Medical Binder" Copyright 2013, Chelsea Makela. All Rights Reserved.

# My Medicine Log

| Medicine Name: | Time to Take: AM/PM | Dose: | With or Without Food? |
|---|---|---|---|
|  |  |  |  |
|  |  |  |  |
|  |  |  |  |
|  |  |  |  |
|  |  |  |  |
|  |  |  |  |
|  |  |  |  |
|  |  |  |  |
|  |  |  |  |
|  |  |  |  |
|  |  |  |  |

"My Medical Binder" Copyright 2013, Chelsea Makela. All Rights Reserved.

# My Medicine Log

| Medicine Name: | Time to Take: AM/PM | Dose: | With or Without Food? |
|---|---|---|---|
| | | | |
| | | | |
| | | | |
| | | | |
| | | | |
| | | | |
| | | | |
| | | | |
| | | | |
| | | | |
| | | | |

# My Medicine Log

| Medicine Name: | Time to Take: AM/PM | Dose: | With or Without Food? |
|---|---|---|---|
|  |  |  |  |
|  |  |  |  |
|  |  |  |  |
|  |  |  |  |
|  |  |  |  |
|  |  |  |  |
|  |  |  |  |
|  |  |  |  |
|  |  |  |  |
|  |  |  |  |
|  |  |  |  |

"My Medical Binder" Copyright 2013, Chelsea Makela. All Rights Reserved.

# My Medicine Log

| Medicine Name: | Time to Take: AM/PM | Dose: | With or Without Food? |
|---|---|---|---|
| | | | |
| | | | |
| | | | |
| | | | |
| | | | |
| | | | |
| | | | |
| | | | |
| | | | |
| | | | |
| | | | |

"My Medical Binder" Copyright 2013, Chelsea Makela. All Rights Reserved.

# My Medicine Log

| Medicine Name: | Time to Take: AM/PM | Dose: | With or Without Food? |
|---|---|---|---|
| | | | |
| | | | |
| | | | |
| | | | |
| | | | |
| | | | |
| | | | |
| | | | |
| | | | |
| | | | |
| | | | |

"My Medical Binder" Copyright 2013, Chelsea Makela. All Rights Reserved.

# My Medicine Log

| Medicine Name: | Time to Take: AM/PM | Dose: | With or Without Food? | |
|---|---|---|---|---|
| | | | | |
| | | | | |
| | | | | |
| | | | | |
| | | | | |
| | | | | |
| | | | | |
| | | | | |
| | | | | |
| | | | | |
| | | | | |

"My Medical Binder" Copyright 2013, Chelsea Makela. All Rights Reserved.

# My Doctors

"My Medical Binder"
Copyright 2013, Chelsea Makela. All Rights Reserved.

Date: _____

Doctor: _____

Opinion: 1st  2nd  3rd  4th  Other: ____

Contact:

Address: _____

Telephone: _____

Fax: _____

Email: _____

**What They Specialize In:**
_____

**Reason for Appointment:**
_____

**Follow Up Date:**
_____

**Appointment Questions:**
_____
_____
_____

**Notes On Appointment:**

"My Medical Binder" Copyright 2013, Chelsea Makela. All Rights Reserved.

Date: _____

Doctor: _____

Opinion: 1st  2nd  3rd  4th  Other: ____

Contact:

Address: _____

Telephone: _____

Fax: _____

Email: _____

**What They Specialize In:**
_____

**Reason for Appointment:**
_____

**Follow Up Date:**
_____

**Appointment Questions:**
_____
_____
_____

**Notes On Appointment:**

"My Medical Binder" Copyright 2013, Chelsea Makela. All Rights Reserved.

Date: _____

Doctor:_____

Opinion: 1st  2nd  3rd  4th  Other: _____

Contact:

Address: _____

Telephone:_____

Fax: _____

Email:_____

**What They Specialize In:**
_____

**Reason for Appointment:**
_____

**Follow Up Date:**
_____

**Appointment Questions:**
_____
_____
_____

**Notes On Appointment:**

"My Medical Binder" Copyright 2013, Chelsea Makela. All Rights Reserved.

Date: _____

Doctor: _____

Opinion: 1st 2nd 3rd 4th Other: _____

Contact:

Address: _____

Telephone: _____

Fax: _____

Email: _____

**What They Specialize In:**

_____

**Reason for Appointment:**

_____

**Follow Up Date:**

_____

**Appointment Questions:**

_____
_____
_____

**Notes On Appointment:**

"My Medical Binder" Copyright 2013, Chelsea Makela. All Rights Reserved.

Date: _____

Doctor:_____

Opinion: 1st  2nd  3rd  4th  Other: _____

Contact:

Address: _____

Telephone:_____

Fax: _____

Email:_____

**What They Specialize In:**

_____

**Reason for Appointment:**

_____

**Follow Up Date:**

_____

**Appointment Questions:**

_____
_____
_____

**Notes On Appointment:**

"My Medical Binder" Copyright 2013, Chelsea Makela. All Rights Reserved.

Date: _____

Doctor: _____

Opinion: 1st  2nd  3rd  4th  Other: _____

Contact:

Address: _____

Telephone: _____

Fax: _____

Email: _____

**What They Specialize In:**

_____

**Reason for Appointment:**

_____

**Follow Up Date:**

_____

**Appointment Questions:**

_____

_____

_____

**Notes On Appointment:**

"My Medical Binder" Copyright 2013, Chelsea Makela. All Rights Reserved.

Date: _____

Doctor: _____

Opinion: 1st  2nd  3rd  4th  Other: _____

Contact:

Address: _____

Telephone: _____

Fax: _____

Email: _____

**What They Specialize In:**

_____

**Reason for Appointment:**

_____

**Follow Up Date:**

_____

**Appointment Questions:**

_____
_____
_____

**Notes On Appointment:**

"My Medical Binder" Copyright 2013, Chelsea Makela. All Rights Reserved.

Date: _____

Doctor: _____

Opinion: 1st  2nd  3rd  4th  Other: _____

Contact:

Address: _____

Telephone: _____

Fax: _____

Email: _____

**What They Specialize In:**

_____

**Reason for Appointment:**

_____

**Follow Up Date:**

_____

**Appointment Questions:**

_____
_____
_____

**Notes On Appointment:**

"My Medical Binder" Copyright 2013, Chelsea Makela. All Rights Reserved.

Date: _____

Doctor: _____

Opinion: 1st  2nd  3rd  4th  Other: _____

Contact:

Address: _____

Telephone: _____

Fax: _____

Email: _____

**What They Specialize In:**

_____

**Reason for Appointment:**

_____

**Follow Up Date:**

_____

**Appointment Questions:**

_____
_____
_____

**Notes On Appointment:**

"My Medical Binder" Copyright 2013, Chelsea Makela. All Rights Reserved.

Date: _____
Doctor: _____
Opinion: 1st  2nd  3rd  4th  Other: _____
Contact:
Address: _____
Telephone: _____
Fax: _____
Email: _____

**What They Specialize In:**
_____

**Reason for Appointment:**
_____

**Follow Up Date:**

_____

**Appointment Questions:**
_____
_____
_____

**Notes On Appointment:**

"My Medical Binder" Copyright 2013, Chelsea Makela. All Rights Reserved.

# Procedures & Treatments I've Received

"My Medical Binder" Copyright 2013, Chelsea Makela. All Rights Reserved.

| Treatment/ Procedure & Doctor: | Type/Dose: | Start & Finish Date(s): |
|---|---|---|
| | | |
| | | |
| | | |
| | | |
| | | |
| | | |
| | | |
| | | |
| | | |

"My Medical Binder" Copyright 2013, Chelsea Makela. All Rights Reserved.

| Treatment/ Procedure & Doctor: | Type/Dose: | Start & Finish Date(s): |
|---|---|---|
| | | |
| | | |
| | | |
| | | |
| | | |
| | | |
| | | |
| | | |
| | | |

"My Medical Binder" Copyright 2013, Chelsea Makela. All Rights Reserved.

| Treatment/ Procedure & Doctor: | Type/Dose: | Start & Finish Date(s): |
|---|---|---|
| | | |
| | | |
| | | |
| | | |
| | | |
| | | |
| | | |
| | | |
| | | |

"My Medical Binder" Copyright 2013, Chelsea Makela. All Rights Reserved.

| Treatment/ Procedure & Doctor: | Type/Dose: | Start & Finish Date(s): |
| --- | --- | --- |
| | | |
| | | |
| | | |
| | | |
| | | |
| | | |
| | | |
| | | |
| | | |

"My Medical Binder" Copyright 2013, Chelsea Makela. All Rights Reserved.

| Treatment/ Procedure & Doctor: | Type/Dose: | Start & Finish Date(s): |
|---|---|---|
| | | |
| | | |
| | | |
| | | |
| | | |
| | | |
| | | |
| | | |
| | | |

"My Medical Binder" Copyright 2013, Chelsea Makela. All Rights Reserved.

# Questions & Notes

"My Medical Binder"
Copyright 2013, Chelsea Makela. All Rights Reserved.

# NOTES

# NOTES

"My Medical Binder" Copyright 2013, Chelsea Makela. All Rights Reserved.

# NOTES

# NOTES

# NOTES

Thank you for purchasing *"My Medical Binder"*. As a child I was diagnosed with cancer and the amount of medical information my parents and I received became impossible to simply just "remember". To help with this my Mom and I created a medical binder that both my parents and I would use to store information given to us by doctors and nurses. We'd also use it to take note of dates, schedules we had and notes on things we wanted to ask or tell doctors. I hope that you find this binder both useful and helpful for storing your medical information and schedule. Thank you for your continued support. To learn more about me and my journey visit my official website:
www.chelseamakela.com
Thank You,
Chelsea Makela
*Creator of "My Medical Binder"*

"My Medical Binder" Copyright 2013, Chelsea Makela. All Rights Reserved.

www.ingramcontent.com/pod-product-compliance
Lightning Source LLC
Chambersburg PA
CBHW050803180526
45159CB00004B/1536